Natural Care Library

VITAMIN E

ANTI-AGING ANTI-OXIDANT

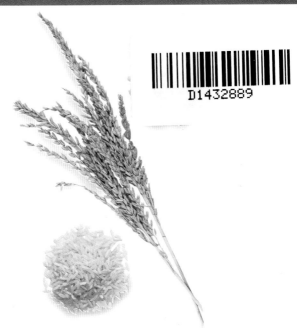

D1432889

By STEPHANIE PEDERSEN

DORLING KINDERSLEY PUBLISHING, INC.

www.dk.com

CONTENTS

VITAMIN BASICS

The word "vitamin" is a relatively new term. The word first appeared in dictionaries in 1912 and was coined to describe the organic substances in food essential for most chemical processes in the body. Before vitamins were discovered, doctors recommended food itself: carrots (rich in vitamin A) to maintain vision, citrus fruit (high in vitamin C) to prevent scurvy, and whole grains and legumes (abundant in vitamin B_1) to ward off beriberi.

Scientists have identified 13 vitamins that are considered essential for health—essential because the body does not manufacture these nutrients itself. In other words, these vitamins must come either from food or from supplements. Essential vitamins are grouped into two categories: fat-soluble and water-soluble.

Essential fat-soluble vitamins include vitamins A, D, E, and K. These are stored in the body's fat to be used as needed. Because the body stockpiles fat-soluble vitamins, it is possible to take too much of one or more of these vitamins, although this rarely occurs. Vitamin overdose can lead to various symptoms, including headaches and irritability.

The essential water-soluble vitamins are C, B, B_1, B_2, B_3, B_5, B_6, B_{12}, folic acid, and biotin. These are not stored in the body: The body uses just what it needs at any given time and excretes the unused amount in the urine.

Two important points about vitamins. Many people believe that if they take nutritional supplements, they won't have to worry about a balanced diet. But vitamins are just that, supplements. It is important to remember that the human body absorbs vitamins from food more readily than from pills. In addition, science is rapidly discovering dozens of health-supportive phytonutrients in food that work with vitamins to promote health—and these phytonutrients are unavailable in pill form.

Another important point to remember when it comes to vitamins is that you can have too much of a good thing. While large amounts of some vitamins are helpful in specific situations, too much may cause side effects that range from the merely annoying (such as dry skin or sleep disturbances) to the truly dangerous (such as liver damage).

HOW TO TAKE VITAMIN SUPPLEMENTS

• Take vitamin supplements with food to increase absorption. Fat-soluble vitamins should be eaten with food containing some fat.

• If you experience nausea within a half-hour after taking a vitamin, you may not have had enough food in your stomach.

• High doses of vitamins should not be taken at one time. For most efficient absorption, space dosages throughout the day.

WHAT IS VITAMIN E?

Vitamin E is one of the most talked-about vitamins in America. And with good reason. It is a powerful antioxidant, responsible for protecting the body from pollutants, chemicals, and rancid fats that create the free radicals which in turn contribute to cancer and break down other nutrients in the body. Vitamin E also protects the heart by preventing cholesterol deposits from forming on artery walls and by strengthening arteries. Additionally, it thins cholesterol-thickened blood so the blood can more easily circulate through the body; this not only aids the heart, but helps prevent and reduce the symptoms of Alzheimer's disease and other dementias. The vitamin is also needed both to produce red blood cells and to extend the life of red blood cells, thus helping to ward off anemia. Vitamin E is necessary, as well, for tissue repair and regeneration—hence its role in wound healing, muscle conditions, and joint diseases. The vitamin even boasts hormone-balancing effects, making it an important nutrient for women with menopausal or menstrual difficulties.

Despite its wide-ranging importance, vitamin E is a recent discovery. It was first identified in 1922 when researchers found that rats fed a limited diet became infertile. However, after receiving wheat germ oil—which happens to be high in vitamin E—the rats became fertile again. When the responsible nutrient was isolated, scientists named it tocopherol, after the Greek words *tokos* and *phero*, which mean "offspring" and "to bear."

Vitamin E is a fat-soluble vitamin that is actually comprised of two families of compounds: the tocopherols (alpha, beta, gamma, delta, epsilon, and zeta) and the tocotrienols (alpha, beta, gamma, and delta). Of all its constituents, alpha-tocopherol, delta-tocopherol, and gamma-tocopherol are the most studied—

although all vitamin E constituents are beneficial.

Unlike the other fat-soluble vitamins—A, D, and K—vitamin E is not effectively stored in the body. After ingestion, it finds its way to the intestines, where it is absorbed along with fat and bile salts—first into the lymphatic system and then into the blood, which carries it to the liver to be used or stored. Over half of any excess may be lost in the feces, but some vitamin E is stored in the fatty tissues and the liver, and to a lesser degree, in the heart, muscles, testes, uterus, adrenal and pituitary glands, and blood. Vitamin E is also partially absorbed through the skin when used as an ointment or oil application.

Vitamin E is found in small amounts in animal foods. Yet it is plant foods that are richest in the vitamin. In fact, the best sources of vitamin E are cold-pressed oils from nuts, seeds, and vegetables. Unfortunately, during the modern refinement and purification of oils, grains, flours, fruits, and vegetables, vitamin E is lost. Interestingly, the byproducts of today's refining processes, which are rich in vitamin E, are used to make vitamin E supplements. Based on the fresh, unprocessed, whole-foods diet of early humans, many authorities feel humans need 200 to 1200 IU (international units) or more of vitamin E daily—quite a bit more than the current RDA (recommeded daily allowances) of 12 to 15 IU. For that reason, throughout the book, a range of vitamin E dosages are offered.

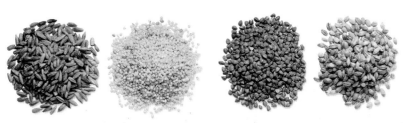

FOOD SOURCES

Food is an important, easily digested source of a wide range of vitamins. The following foods are particularly rich in vitamin E:

- Almonds
- Avocados
- Brown rice
- Cold-pressed nut and vegetable oils
- Cornmeal
- Desiccated liver
- Dried beans
- Dulce
- Greens (all kinds)
- Hazelnuts
- Kelp
- Oatmeal
- Organ meats
- Soybeans
- Sweet potatoes
- Sunflower seeds
- Walnuts
- Wheat germ
- Whole wheat flour

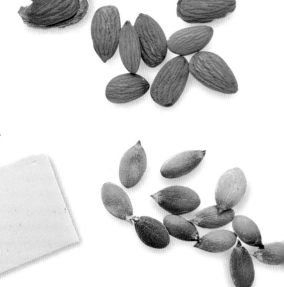

NATURAL OR SYNTHETIC?

What kind of vitamin E is best for you—natural or synthetic? It seems that the natural variety is better absorbed in the body. Japanese researchers gave seven healthy women, ages 21 to 37, supplements of natural and synthetic vitamin E. They found that the bioavailability of natural vitamin E was substantially greater than that of synthetic vitamin E. If you're having difficulty separating what's natural from what's synthetic, look for "d-alpha-tocopherol with a mix of natural tocopherols" on the label; "dl-alpha-tocopherol" indicates synthetic vitamin E.

HOW MUCH DO I TAKE?

How many times have you stood in front of the vitamin shelves in your local health food store or pharmacy and compared labels? And how many times have you wondered why one brand offers 60 mg of vitamin C when another boasts 750 mg of vitamin C? Or why another product has 180 mcg of folate when a competing brand features 400 mcg of the same nutrient? And perhaps more importantly, which one is better? When it comes to dosages, there is no magic number. Minimum requirements for nutrients are set by a government board called The Food and Nutrition Board of the National Research Council. These numbers are the recommended daily allowances (RDA) needed to avoid nutritional deficiency diseases such as beriberi, rickets, or scurvy. However, many researchers, medical experts, and health authorities believe that the body needs much higher levels of vitamins for optimum health. And in the presence of illness, pollution, prescription medication, or stress, the body may need still higher levels. For this reason, throughout this book, we suggest a range of vitamin dosages. To determine the best level for you, consult your physician.

SPECIAL NEEDS

While a daily dose of 12 to 15 IU of vitamin E is recommended, the following individuals have increased needs for vitamin E:

• Smokers. Cigarette, cigar, and pipe smoking deplete the body of vitamin E.

• Alcoholics. Alcohol reduces levels of vitamin E in the body.

• Individuals who eat only cooked fruits or processed fruits and vegetables. Canning, cooking, and freezing break down the vitamin E in foods.

• Individuals who live in polluted environments or who are exposed to secondhand smoke. Pollution and secondhand smoke stress the immune system, thus depleting vitamin E levels in the body.

• The elderly. With age comes a reduced ability to absorb vitamin E.

• Individuals who are ill or who are scheduled for or have recently had surgery. The body uses increased levels of vitamin E to recover from illness and surgery.

• Individuals who eat fried and deep-fried foods daily. When oil is heated to a certain temperature, free radicals are created. When consumed, these free radicals are believed to contribute to cancer. Vitamin E's antioxidant actions help neutralize these free radicals.

• Individuals on birth control pills or other types of hormone therapy. Estrogen depletes vitamin E stores in the body.

VITAMIN E DEFICIENCY

SYMPTOMS of VITAMIN E DEFICIENCY
- Anemia
- Dementia
- Fatigue
- Infertility
- Joint pain
- Menstrual problems
- Muscle pain
- Neuromuscular impairment

TOO MUCH OF A GOOD THING
Although it is fat-soluble, vitamin E is considered nontoxic because it is not harmful except in extremely high doses. Excessive vitamin E supplementation may cause the following symptoms in some individuals:

- Abdominal bloating
- Diarrhea
- Dizziness
- Excessive iron absorption
- Flatulence
- Nausea
- Reduced clotting ability
- Reduced vitamin A absorption
- Reduced vitamin D absorption
- Reduced vitamin K absorption
- Stomach upset

RETHINKING MEDICATION

ANTIBIOTICS: ARE THEY ESSENTIAL?

A recent report published in the *Journal of the American Medical Association* stated that even though antibiotics provide little help for colds, upper respiratory tract infections, and bronchitis, doctors still prescribe antibiotics for these conditions. Why? In part, because patients expect their doctors to give them some kind of medication, and many physicians find it easier to oblige than take time out to explain how antibiotics do and don't work. Americans are so enamored of antibiotics that doctors write over 12 million antibiotic prescriptions annually. To learn more about the dangers of antibiotic abuse, contact the Centers For Disease Control and Prevention, 404-332-4555.

PENICILLIN BY THE POUND

Since penicillin's debut in 1941, antibiotic production has shot up from 2 million pounds in 1954 to more than 50 million pounds in 1997. Where is all this medication going? Half of the antibiotics produced annually are prescribed for people; the rest are mixed into livestock feed and used as fertilizers for agricultural crops. The downside to this free-flowing penicillin? New, strong, antibiotic-resistant strains of bacteria.

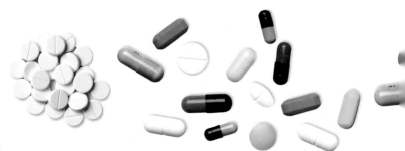

WAIT! BEFORE YOU TAKE THAT PILL . . .
Before asking your doctor for an antibiotic, ask yourself the following questions:

✔ Is my condition caused by bacteria? If not, antibiotics will not work.

✔ Are antibiotics necessary for recovery? If the infection will go away on its own, consider forgoing antibiotics.

✔ Are there alternatives to antibiotics? If herbal or other natural remedies can fight off the infection, consider using one or more of them.

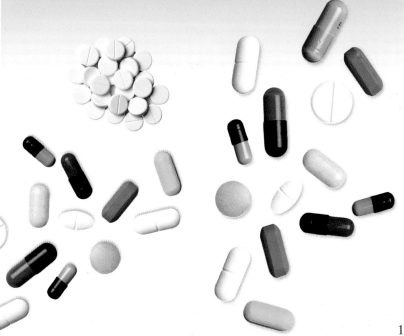

CONDITIONS AND DOSES

ALZHEIMER'S DISEASE

❏ **Symptoms:** How many times have you heard someone call Alzheimer's disease "old-timer's disease"? The mistake is a natural one, considering Alzheimer's primarily hits older adults. While the disease can strike people in their 40s or 50s, it most commonly affects those aged 65 and older. In fact, about every one in ten people over the age of 65 is diagnosed with Alzheimer's and studies show that over 4 million Americans have the disease.

Alzheimer's is an incurable disease that destroys brain cells—usually those of the cerebral cortex—causing dementia. Symptoms appear progressively, usually in this order: forgetfulness, shortening of attention span, disintegration of personality, disorientation, memory loss, confusion, restlessness, inability to read, wandering, lack of patience, loss of impulse control, inappropriate behavior, aggressiveness, irritability, cursing, incoordination, delusions, hallucinations, loss of language, lack of bladder and bowel control, and inability to feed oneself.

Currently, there is no diagnostic test for Alzheimer's; the most foolproof test for the disease is an autopsy to examine brain tissue. That said, physicians can make an accurate diagnosis in up to 90 percent of all cases after a careful medical history and physical examination. It's not known exactly what causes Alzheimer's. Some researchers believe it is an inflammatory response to infection; others blame it on free radicals, environmental toxins, or lack of blood flow to the brain. Whatever the culprit, genetics is often a factor.

❒ **How Vitamin E Can Help:** Right now there is no cure for Alzheimer's disease. However, vitamin E has been shown by several studies to be an effective companion therapy to other herbal and nutritional treatments in delaying the onset of the disease or lessening its severity. Vitamin E is an antioxidant that helps transport oxygen to the brain cells and protect them from free radical damage. It is also an anticoagulant that thins thickened blood, making it easier for red blood cells to reach the brain. Furthermore, autopsies show that Alzheimer's victims are found to have radically reduced levels of vitamin E in their bodies.

❒ **Dosages:** As a preventative or companion therapy to conventional treatment, take 10 to 200 mg of vitamin E three times daily with meals. In addition, consume daily servings of foods rich in vitamin E, such as avocados, brown rice, dark green leafy vegetables, nuts, oatmeal, seeds, soybeans, and wheat germ.

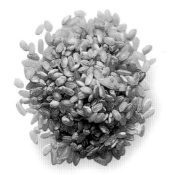
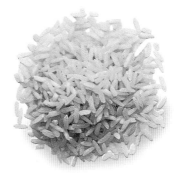

CONDITIONS AND DOSES

ANEMIA

❏ **Symptoms:** Anemia, also called iron-deficiency anemia, occurs when there is not enough iron in the body. Without the proper amount of this mineral, the body cannot produce adequate amounts of hemoglobin. Why does this matter? Hemoglobin is responsible for carrying tissue-nourishing oxygen from the lungs to every part of the body. Without oxygen, the body cannot function properly. A low-iron diet, heavy monthly menstrual flow, pregnancy, lead poisoning, recent blood loss, or poor iron absorption by the body can all lead to anemia. Initial signs are so mild they often go unnoticed: Greater-than-usual fatigue or slight pallor are common symptoms. Later on, the heart rate may grow faster and the sufferer may become winded more easily than usual.

❏ **How Vitamin E Can Help:** Two of vitamin E's functions are to help form new red blood cells and maintain the health of existing red blood cells, allowing them to live "a long life." While vitamin E alone cannot cure anemia, its essential role in maintaining a healthy blood supply makes it a helpful companion therapy.

❏ **Dosages:** Take 10 to 200 mg of vitamin E three times daily with meals. In addition, consume daily servings of foods rich in vitamin E, such as avocados, brown rice, dark green leafy vegetables, nuts, oatmeal, seeds, soybeans, and wheat germ.

BLOOD BOOSTER
Want to know just how important vitamin E is to a healthy blood supply? In one study, male adults were fed a diet containing no more than 5 IU of vitamin E daily for several years. Routine tests found that the test subjects' hemoglobin levels were in what researchers call "a normal, slightly low range." Furthermore, data showed that the red blood cells of these subjects were being destroyed about 8 to 10 percent faster than the red blood cells of the control group subjects, who were getting higher levels of vitamin E from their diets.

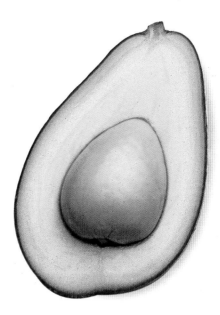

CONDITIONS AND DOSES

ASTHMA

❏ **Symptoms:** Asthma is an inflammation of the airways. It is caused by an allergic reaction and is estimated to affect between 10 million and 14 million Americans. Although not all sufferers are allergic to the same substances, some common triggers are animal dander, dust mites, mold spores, and pollen. When a trigger is inhaled, the body's antibodies react with the allergen, producing allergen-suppressing histamine and other chemicals. Also, chest muscles constrict, the bronchial lining swells, and the body creates more mucus, thus causing breathing difficulties, coughing (sometimes accompanied by mucus), painless tightness in the chest, and wheezing.

❏ **How Vitamin E Can Help:** While vitamin E cannot cure asthma, it has been shown to help prevent attacks and lessen symptoms during an attack. How does it work? Vitamin E is an antioxidant. This is important because asthma attacks frequently occur when the lungs are under stress from allergens. These allergens produce oxidants that weaken the smooth muscle wall of the bronchi. Vitamin E can help squelch the oxidants, preventing them from weakening the lungs and provoking an asthma attack.

❏ **Dosages:** As a preventative or companion therapy to conventional treatment, take 10 to 200 mg of vitamin E three times daily with meals. In addition, consume daily servings of foods rich in vitamin E, as avocados, brown rice, dark green leafy vegetables, nuts, oatmeal, seeds, soybeans, and wheat germ.

MISERY HAS COMPANY

If you suffer from asthma, you're not alone. According to the American Lung Association, since 1982, the prevalence of asthma in the United States increased by 49 percent; among children under age 18, the rate rose 78.6 percent. More breathtaking statistics: More than 4,000 people die each year from serious asthma attacks.

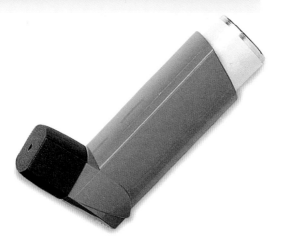

CONDITIONS AND DOSES

CANCER

❒ **Symptoms:** Cancer occurs when cells begin growing abnormally, forming malignant tumors. These malignant tumors can appear in the breast, the bones, the throat, the brain, the stomach—actually, in almost any area of the body. But why do cells begin acting strangely in the first place? It's believed that exposure to carcinogens causes free radical damage to the cells, which in turn prompts cells to mutate. Common carcinogens include cigarette smoke, fatty foods, industrial chemicals, insecticides, nuclear radiation, pesticides used on food, polluted air, and UV (ultraviolet) light. While cancer symptoms vary widely depending on what part of the body is affected, general signs include blood in the urine or stool, fatigue, hoarseness, indigestion, nagging cough, sores that do not heal, thickening somewhere in the body, and unexplained weight loss.

❒ **How Vitamin E Can Help:** While vitamin E cannot wipe out established cancers, it is a powerful antioxidant. In other words, it has the power to stop free radical damage at a cellular level, thus stopping cancerous cell mutations before they start. As proof of vitamin E's cancer-fighting power, several epidemiological studies have shown that individuals who eat large amounts of foods rich in vitamin E each day have significantly lower cancer rates than individuals who eat foods containing little or no vitamin E.

❏ **Dosages:** As a preventative or companion therapy to conventional cancer treatment, take 50 to 200 mg of vitamin E three times daily with meals. In addition, consume daily servings of foods rich in vitamin E, such as avocados, brown rice, dark green leafy vegetables, nuts, oatmeal, seeds, soybeans, and wheat germ.

CANCER FACTS

• In the United States, nearly one person dies of cancer every minute.

• According to the American Cancer Society, the incidence of cancer is highest in Florida, West Virginia, Pennsylvania, and Arkansas, respectively. It is lowest in New Mexico, Hawaii, Utah, and Alaska.

• There are more than 100 different varieties of cancer.

• People with breast cancer have been found to have lower-than-normal levels of vitamin E and the mineral selenium—two important antioxidants that neutralize free radicals.

• African-Americans have the highest incidence of prostate cancer, while Asian-Americans have the lowest.

• An estimated 60,000 Americans develop some type of skin cancer each year, and over 10,000 individuals die from the disease annually.

• It is believed that intestinal cancer takes up to 20 years to develop.

• The single most avoidable cancer risk is smoking.

• People whose mothers smoked during pregnancy are about 50 percent more likely than children of nonsmoking mothers to develop cancer later in life.

Conditions and Doses

CORONARY ARTERY DISEASE

❒ **Symptoms:** Coronary artery disease accounts for about one in two American deaths each year. The disease progresses slowly over the course of years and even decades, but its impact can be instantaneous: In nearly one-third of all cases, death occurs without any previous warning of disease. Indeed, some people have no symptoms, while others may experience chest pain, constriction or a sense of heaviness in the chest, fatigue, pallor, shortness of breath, swelling in the ankles, and weakness. Coronary artery disease occurs when cholesterol deposits build up on coronary artery walls. These special blood vessels provide oxygen and nutrients to the muscles of the heart. When they are unable to deliver adequate blood flow, however, the heart muscle begins to weaken, leading to angina (chest pain), congestive heart failure, and heart attack. When it comes to causes, a high-fat diet is most often implicated, although heredity, stress, inactivity, smoking, and alcoholism are also culprits.

❒ **How Vitamin E Can Help:** Several studies have found that vitamin E is an effective treatment and preventative for coronary artery disease. The vitamin works in several ways: by decreasing the liver's production of cholesterol, thus lowering the amount of cholesterol circulating in the blood; and by keeping cholesterol from oxidizing and depositing on arterial walls. Vitamin E is also an effective anticoagulant, keeping blood thin so it can easily pass though clogged arteries.

❏ **Dosages:** As a preventative or companion therapy to conventional treatment, take 10 to 200 mg of vitamin E three times daily with meals. In addition, consume daily servings of foods rich in vitamin E, such as avocados, brown rice, dark green leafy vegetables, nuts, oatmeal, seeds, soybeans, and wheat germ. **Note:** If you are currently on anticoagulant medication, consult with a physician before taking more than 100 mg of vitamin E daily.

HOW MUCH VITAMIN E IS ENOUGH?

While the RDA for vitamin E is set at 12 IU for women and 15 IU for men and pregnant women, many experts feel that the IU should be much higher. As proof, researchers point to studies such as a recent double-blind, placebo-controlled intervention trial that showed a significant decrease in nonfatal heart attacks in high-risk subjects (individuals with high cholesterol and/or high blood pressure, smokers, and subjects with a history of heart attacks) who consumed either 400 IU or 800 IU of vitamin E supplements per day. In comparison, a Finnish clinical trial did not observe any benefit against heart disease when vitamin E was given at a more modest daily dose of 50 IU to long-term, heavy smokers.

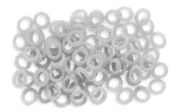 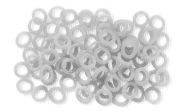

CONDITIONS AND DOSES

HIGH BLOOD CHOLESTEROL

❐ **Symptoms:** High blood cholesterol refers to high levels of fat in the blood. Blame the condition on a fatty diet, heredity, alcoholism, smoking, sedentary lifestyle, or a combination thereof. Whatever the cause, the condition is dangerous. Gummy in texture, fat thickens blood and gets stuck on artery walls, thus increasing one's risk of coronary artery disease, heart attack, and stroke. Symptoms can include chest pain, lethargy, pallor, and shortness of breath. However, the condition is often asymptomatic; many individuals learn they have high cholesterol only after a routine blood test.

❐ **How Vitamin E Can Help:** Vitamin E is a proven preventative treatment against high blood cholesterol, as well as an effective companion therapy for the disease when used with herbal or prescription medications. The vitamin works by decreasing the liver's production of cholesterol, lowering the amount of cholesterol circulating in the blood, and by keeping cholesterol from oxidizing and depositing on arterial walls. Vitamin E is also an effective anticoagulant, keeping cholesterol-thick blood thin so it can easily pass though arteries.

❏ **Dosages:** As a preventative or companion therapy to conventional treatment, take 10 to 200 mg of vitamin E three times daily with meals. In addition, consume daily servings of foods rich in vitamin E, such as avocados, brown rice, dark green leafy vegetables, nuts, oatmeal, seeds, soybeans, and wheat germ. **Note:** If you are currently on anticoagulant medication, consult with a physician before taking more than 100 mg of vitamin E daily.

NUTS TO YOU

The Nurses Health Study, a long-term study by Brigham and Women's Hospital in Boston and the Harvard School of Public Health, has been monitoring the health of over 87,000 nurses. Researchers found that individuals who ate more than five ounces of nuts rich in vitamin E per week had one-third fewer heart attacks than those who rarely or never ate nuts. Preliminary results from a companion study, the Physicians Health Study, indicate that eating nuts may provide the same health benefits to men. But wait, there's more: Another study of 40,000 postmenopausal women found that those who ate the most nuts reduced their risk of coronary artery disease by 60 percent.

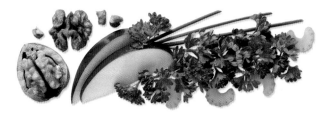

CONDITIONS AND DOSES

HYPERTENSION

❏ **Symptoms:** Hypertension, more commonly known as high blood pressure, is a condition in which blood travels through the arteries at higher-than-normal pressure. This increased blood flow literally wears out the blood vessels, heart, and kidneys and can lead to premature death. What causes hypertension? Cigarettes, alcohol, some medications, and certain illnesses can elevate blood pressure. But by far the most common cause of hypertension is clogged arteries from a high-fat diet. When blood vessels are blocked with fatty deposits, the heart must work harder to move the same amount of blood through them. This in turn increases the pressure at which the blood is pumped. Unfortunately, hypertension is symptomless, leaving many individuals unaware that they even suffer from the condition—until it's too late.

❏ **How Vitamin E Can Help:** Vitamin E cannot cure hypertension. Vitamin E helps in tissue repair, so what it can do is help rebuild and strengthen artery walls that have been weakened by the constant stress of blood flowing through at high pressure. Vitamin E also thins cholesterol-thickened blood so that it passes more easily through the arteries. The heart does not have to work as hard to pump thinner blood through the arteries, thus creating lower blood pressure.

❏ **Dosages:** As a preventative or companion therapy to conventional treatment, take 10 to 200 mg of vitamin E three times daily with meals. In addition, consume daily servings of foods rich in vitamin E, such as avocados, brown rice, dark green leafy vegetables, nuts, oatmeal, seeds, soybeans, and wheat germ. **Note:** If you are currently on anticoagulant medication, consult with a physician before taking more than 100 mg of vitamin E daily.

TIME IS OF THE ESSENCE
According to at least one study, when it comes to vitamin E, the length of time a person has taken vitamin E supplements may be just as important as the amount taken (and maybe even more important). From 1974 to 1985, researcher Richard Passwater studied 17,894 persons between the ages of 50 and 98. His findings? Taking 400 IU or more of vitamin E daily for ten years strongly reduced the incidence of heart disease prior to eighty years of age. In fact, it reduced the rate of heart disease to less than ten percent of the normal rate. Among persons taking vitamin E over ten years, only four suffered from heart disease out of a total of 2,508. According to Passwater, a sample of that size would ordinarily have approximately 836 persons who would have suffered from heart disease. Interestingly, Passwater found that those who took 1200 IU of vitamin E daily for four years also had a dramatic decrease in heart disease incidence, though not as strong as those taking the lower dose for a longer period of time. The conclusion? The longer one takes vitamin E, the longer one is protected against the causes of heart disease.

CONDITIONS AND DOSES

CERVICAL DYSPLASIA

❒ **Symptoms:** Sometimes, a Pap test will show a precancerous cell. If this happens to you, the medical world will diagnose you as having cervical dysplasia. The good news is that cervical dysplasia often disappears on its own. The bad news is it can stick around and lead to cancer some years later. Cervical dysplasia is an asymptomatic condition found most often in women between the ages of 25 and 35. It has been linked to sexually transmitted diseases, such as the human papillomavirus (HPV), which causes genital warts. Infection by sexually transmitted organisms may be accompanied by oxidants, which can damage cervical cell DNA. Eventually, this cellular damage can lead to cancer.

❒ **How Vitamin E Can Help:** Recent research has found that vitamin E can prevent cervical cells from becoming precancerous. The vitamin is a powerful antioxidant, which prevents infected cervical cells from being attacked by cancer-causing oxidants.

❒ **Dosages:** Take 50 to 100 mg of vitamin E three times daily with meals. In addition, consume daily servings of foods rich in vitamin E, such as avocados, brown rice, dark green leafy vegetables, nuts, oatmeal, seeds, soybeans, and wheat germ.

CERVICAL DYSPLASIA AND VITAMIN E

Researchers at the Lublin Medical Academy in Poland evaluated 168 female patients with normal Pap smears who had not been infected by the human papillomavirus and compared the results to 228 patients with cervical dysplasia who were infected with the human papillomavirus. Members of the second group showed significantly lower levels of vitamin E in their blood than members of the first group.

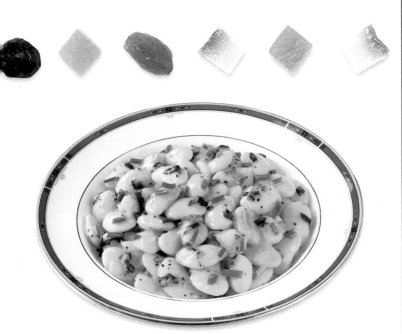

CONDITIONS AND DOSES

ESTROGEN FACTS

• The most prescribed drug in the United States is estrogen, the female sex hormone.

• Some 10 million women in the United States—about one-fourth of those at or past menopause—regularly take artificial estrogen supplements, with or without additional supplements of progesterone (the other female sex hormone).

• It is believed that one-fifth of women who are prescribed estrogen never fill their prescription.

• A recent survey has found that one-third of women prescribed estrogen quit taking it within nine months, and more than half stop within a year.

• Women's bones slowly begin to lose minerals and become less dense even before menopause. Estrogen supplements have been proven to reduce the bone loss associated with osteoporosis. Unless a woman is taking estrogen, she has about a one-in-four chance of developing serious osteoporosis.

• A study of 240,000 women sponsored by the American Cancer Society found that women who took estrogen for at least six years had a 40-percent increased risk of contracting ovarian cancer, a cancer that is frequently fatal.

• Various studies have suggested that estrogen use increases a woman's' risk of breast cancer by as much as 30 percent.

• Statistics show that women who take estrogen are 40 percent less likely to develop Alzheimer's disease than individuals who don't take the hormone. Furthermore, the longer an individual takes estrogen, the more their risk is reduced.

• Estrogen replacement seems to help prevent heart disease in older women. Without estrogen replacement, a woman's' risk of heart attack becomes equal to a man's within 15 years of menopause.

• A report from a ten year study of 48,470 nurses—one of the largest studies to date—found that estrogen use reduced the risk of major coronary disease and fatal cardiovascular disease by half.

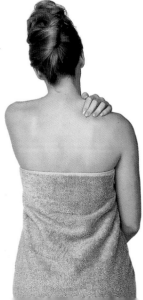

CONDITIONS AND DOSES

FIBROCYSTIC DISEASE

❏ **Symptoms:** Benign breast disease, chronic cystic mastitis, lumpy breasts, and mammary dysplasia are all names for fibrocystic disease, a condition characterized by one or more lumps in one or both breasts. These lumps may or may not be painful and may be accompanied by greenish or straw-colored discharge from the nipples. Unlike malignant tumors, these benign lumps are actually cysts, fluid-filled sacs that tend to get bigger toward the end of the menstrual cycle, when the body retains more fluid. Some cysts can be tiny, others can be the size of an egg. It isn't known exactly what causes fibrocystic disease, although an imbalance of ovarian hormones is believed to play a role. The disease occurs mainly in women between the ages of 25 and 50 and usually disappears with menopause.

❏ **How Vitamin E Can Help:** Several studies have shown that vitamin E is useful in shrinking or eliminating the cysts associated with fibrocystic disease. Vitamin E has been found by researchers to stabilize imbalanced hormone levels, the ostensible cause of fibrocystic disease.

❏ **Dosage:** Take 50 to 100 mg of vitamin E three times daily with meals. In addition, consume daily servings of foods rich in vitamin E, such as avocados, brown rice, dark green leafy vegetables, nuts, oatmeal, seeds, soybeans, and wheat germ.

LIMIT CHEMICAL EXPOSURE

It's nearly impossible to avoid all chemical toxins in today's world. There's ammonia in cleaning products, chlorine in the water, lead in old paint and pipes, dibromochloropropane in pesticides, carbon monoxide from auto exhaust, and toluene, trichloroethylene, and formaldehyde from printers, photocopiers, and fax machines. Many of these toxins have been linked to allergies, breathing problems, cancer, headaches, infertility, lethargy, lung conditions, reduced attention span, and violence. Ideas for lessening toxins include using environmentally sound dry cleaning, drinking filtered water, purchasing (or making) natural cleansers, limiting the amount of driving you do, and adding a few chemical-filtering plants such as dracaena, chrysanthemum, and weeping fig (ficus) to your home.

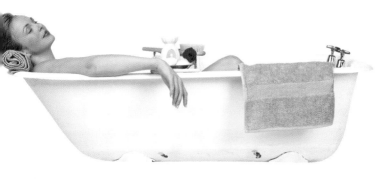

CONDITIONS AND DOSES

MENOPAUSE

❏ **Symptoms:** Menopause is not an illness but a natural condition that occurs when the ovaries no longer produce enough estrogen to stimulate the linings of the uterus and vagina properly. Simply put, menopause is when women no longer menstruate or get pregnant. It generally occurs somewhere between the ages of 40 and 60. One of the most famous signs of menopause is the hot flash, a sudden reddening of the face accompanied by a feeling of intense warmth. Other common symptoms include depressed mood, fluid retention, headache, insomnia, irritability, nervousness, night sweats, painful intercourse, rapid heart beat, susceptibility to bladder problems, thinning of vaginal tissues, vaginal dryness, and weight gain. It should be noted that some women experience few symptoms, while still other encounter none at all.

❏ **How Vitamin E Can Help:** The traditional "remedy" for menopause is hormone replacement therapy. This optional treatment uses synthetic hormones to elevate progesterone and estrogen to their premenopausal levels. Vitamin E is helpful regardless of whether one undergoes or forgoes hormone replacement therapy. Research has shown that the vitamin both diminishes hot flashes and vaginal dryness. It is believed that vitamin E also boasts hormone-regulating effects. By balancing out-of-kilter hormonal levels, theoretically the vitamin helps relieve menopausal symptoms.

❐ **Dosages:** With your physician's okay—and providing you are not currently taking any blood-thinning medication—take 10 to 200 mg of vitamin E three times daily with meals. Vitamin E oil can be used topically up to twice a day to help treat thinning vaginal tissue and vaginal dryness. In addition, consume daily servings of foods rich in vitamin E, such as avocados, brown rice, dark green leafy vegetables, nuts, oatmeal, seeds, soybeans, and wheat germ.

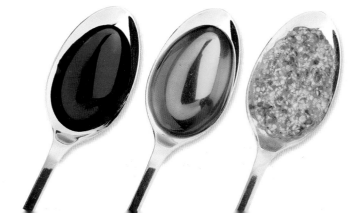

CONDITIONS AND DOSES

PREMENSTRUAL SYNDROME

❏ **Symptoms:** Premenstrual syndrome, popularly known as PMS, is a predictable pattern of physical and emotional changes that occur in some women just before menstruation. Symptoms range from barely noticeable to extreme and can include abdominal swelling, anxiety, bloating, breast soreness, clumsiness, depressed mood, difficulty concentrating, fatigue, fluid retention, headaches, irritability, lethargy, skin eruptions, sleep disturbances, swollen hands and feet, and weight gain. While it is not known exactly what causes the condition, theories include hormonal, nutritional, and psychological factors.

❏ **How Vitamin E Can Help:** Vitamin E is a popular nutritional therapy for PMS. One study reported in the *Journal of Reproductive Medicine* found that the vitamin effectively reduced breast soreness, difficulty concentrating, headaches, and irritability. It is not known exactly how the vitamin affects PMS; one theory is that vitamin E has hormone-regulating effects and thus normalizes hormonal levels.

❏ **Dosages:** As both a preventative and treatment, take 10 to 200 mg of vitamin E three times daily with meals. In addition, consume daily servings of foods rich in vitamin E, such as avocados, brown rice, dark green leafy vegetables, nuts, oatmeal, seeds, soybeans, and wheat germ.

FERTILITY AID?

Infertility is defined as the inability to conceive after a full year of unprotected intercourse. The problem can lie with the male (up to 40 percent of all cases) or female (up to 60 percent of all cases). Although medical measures—fertility drugs, in vitro fertilization, donor eggs or sperm—can increase the chance of conceiving, medical intervention is costly, physically invasive, and time consuming. The alternative? Many researchers claim that vitamin E has helped men and women become fertile in the presence of unexplained infertility. Several small studies—including one of the earliest observations of the physiological effects of vitamin E deficiency—have linked vitamin E and reproductive health. In pregnant female animals deficient in vitamin E, fetuses died; in males, the testes became atrophied. Indeed, vitamin E is stored in large amounts in the female and male reproductive organs. Furthermore, the vitamin's scientific name, tocopherol, is taken from the words *tokos* and *phero*, the Greek words for "offspring" and "to bear." But does any of this mean vitamin E can make an infertile person fertile? Unfortunately, no large-scale study has been done on the subject. Right now, the medical establishment views vitamin E's fertility ability as anecdotal.

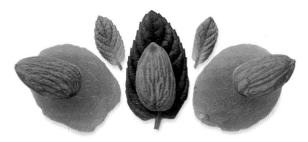

CONDITIONS AND DOSES

RHEUMATOID ARTHRITIS

❐ **Symptoms:** Rheumatoid arthritis is an autoimmune disease in which the body's immune system attacks itself. Though the ailment is not well understood, it is believed that an unidentified virus stimulates the body to attack its own joints. Symptoms include pain and swelling in the smaller joints of hands and feet, overall aching and/or stiffness after periods of inactivity, and local fever in affected joints.

❐ **How Vitamin E Can Help:** Vitamin E is a helpful companion therapy that can be used in conjunction with other vitamins, herbs, and medications. The vitamin is a powerful antioxidant that protects joints from damage by free radicals, thus increasing joint mobility. Moreover, regular intake of vitamin E has been shown in small studies to lessen rheumatoid arthritis pain.

❐ **Dosages:** Take 10 to 100 mg of vitamin E three times daily with meals. In addition, consume daily servings of foods rich in vitamin E, such as avocados, brown rice, dark green leafy vegetables, nuts, oatmeal, seeds, soybeans, and wheat germ.

IT'S ALL IN THE DOSAGE

An eight-year study of 87,245 nurses at Brigham and Women's Hospital in Boston found that women who got more than 100 IU of vitamin E a day had 36 percent fewer heart attacks than those who consumed less than 30 IU a day.

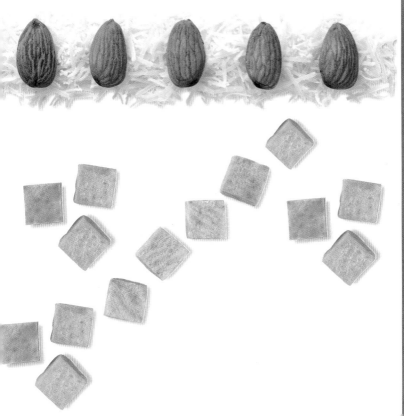

CONDITIONS AND DOSES

SUNBURNS

❒ **Symptoms:** First-degree to second-degree burns caused by the sun's ultraviolet rays, leave the affected area red, inflamed, tender, painful, and sometimes blistered. The amount of sun exposure that can cause a burn—also known as ultraviolet skin damage—depends on the amount of protective melanin an individual has in his or her skin, atmospheric conditions, the geographical location, and the time of day.

❒ **How Vitamin E Can Help:** Vitamin E cannot prevent sunburn—only sun avoidance, sunblock, and/or protective clothing can do that. What vitamin E can do, according to several new American and German studies, is to help bolster the skin's internal resistance to ultraviolet rays. Studies have found that vitamin E can help reduce the incidence of sunburn 10 to 20 percent. Vitamin E is a powerful antioxidant that can help prevent free radical damage at a cellular level, thus halting a large amount of ultraviolet damage before it starts.

❒ **Dosages:** As a preventative, take 50 to 200 mg of vitamin E three times daily with meals. In addition, consume daily servings of foods rich in vitamin E, such as avocados, brown rice, dark green leafy vegetables, nuts, oatmeal, seeds, soybeans, and wheat germ.

BLOCK THAT SCAR

Ouch! You just cut yourself! Chances are, someone—a mom, friend, coworker, passerby—has told you to put vitamin E oil on the wound to speed healing and decrease the chance of scarring. Does it work? While many physicians question vitamin E's effectiveness as a wound-healer, several small studies have found that vitamin E does facilitate healing. After all, vitamin E is necessary for tissue generation, so it makes sense that it could help mend wounds. To try it yourself, wait a day or two for the cut to close, then gently rub vitamin E oil onto the affected area. Repeat up to twice a day. Puncture capsules of the vitamin and squeeze out the contents for application; or head to the health food store, where you can purchase a small bottle of vitamin E oil.

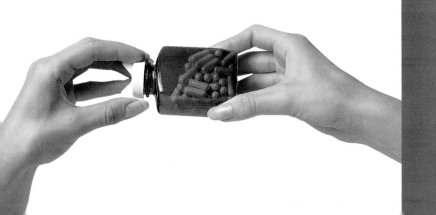

ALTERNATIVE HEALTH STRATEGIES

Herbs, vitamins, minerals—of course these contribute to good health. But creating general well-being involves more than simply taking supplements. Good health has to do with various quality-of-life issues that can aggravate or cause stress, thus harming health. Here are some additional ways to help keep yourself well.

Improve Your Eating Habits

Here are the five main eating strategies people follow; consider finding the most healthful one that works with your lifestyle.

- OMNIVOROUS
- PISCATORIAL
- MACROBIOTIC
- VEGAN
- VEGETARIAN

Get More Exercise

Whether it's walking or weightlifting, exercise can help you feel better. Try any of these types:

- STRETCHING
- AEROBICS
- STRENGTH TRAINING

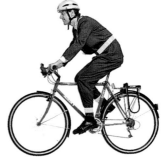

Simple Ways To Ease Stress

In addition to exercise and healthful eating, here are some more techniques—old and new—for easing stress and increasing relaxation.

- GET ENOUGH SLEEP
- MEDITATE REGULARLY
- GIVE UP JUNK FOOD
- ADOPT A PET
- SURROUND YOURSELF WITH SUPPORTIVE PEOPLE
- LIMIT YOUR EXPOSURE TO CHEMICALS
- TAKE YOUR VITAMINS
- ENJOY YOURSELF

ONE-MINUTE STRESS REDUCER

Stress is one of the top health hazards we face today. Unfortunately, it's impossible to go through life without the irritations that make us tense. Fortunately, there *is* something you can do to minimize their power to aggravate you. It's called deep breathing, and it can be done anywhere and anytime you need to calm and center yourself. Here's how to do it:

1. Inhale deeply through your nose.
2. Hold your breath for up to three seconds, then exhale through your mouth.
3. Continue as needed.

Deep breathing pulls a person's attention away from a given stressor and refocuses it on his or her breath. This type of breathing is not only comforting (thanks to its rhythmic quality), but also has been shown to lower rapid pulse and shallow respiration—two temporary symptoms of stress.

GET MOVING

Ask medical experts to name one stay-young strategy and there's a good chance "exercise" will be the answer. And with good reason. Exercise, whether a gentle walk around the block or a full-tilt weight-lifting session, strengthens the heart, lowers the body's resting heart rate, builds muscles, boosts circulation to the body and the brain, revs up the metabolism, and burns calories. All of which can keep a person looking and feeling his or her best. To be effective, exercise must be performed several times a week. Aim for at least three sessions. However, there's more than one kind of exercise. For optimum health, try a combination of aerobic exercise and strength training. And don't forget to stretch before and after each workout!

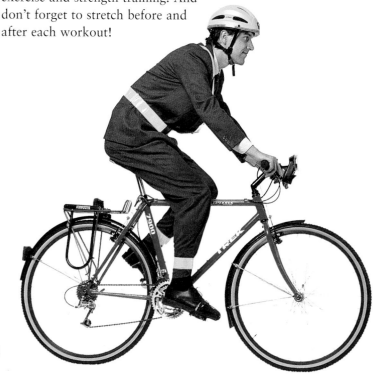

STRETCHING

❒ **What It Is:** Any movement that stretches muscles. Examples include bending at the waist and touching the toes, sitting with legs outstretched in front of you, and rolling your neck. Stretch for eight to twelve minutes before every workout and again after you exercise.

❒ **Why It's Important:** Muscles act like springs. If a muscle is short and tight, it loses the ability to absorb shock. The less shock a muscle can absorb, the more strain there is on the joints. Thus, stretching maintains flexibility, which in turn prevents injuries. Because we often lose our regular range of motion with age, stretching is especially important for older adults to prevent sprains, strains and falls.

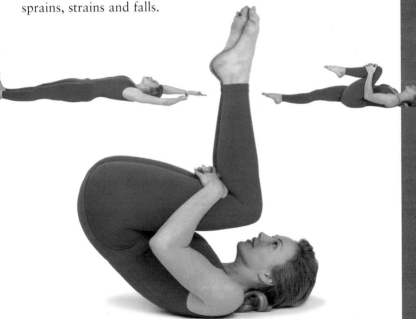

GET MOVING

AEROBICS

❐ **What It Is:** Any activity that uses large muscle groups, is maintained continuously for 15 minutes or more, and is rhythmic in nature. Examples include aerobic dance, jogging, skating, and walking. Ideally, you should aim for three to six aerobic workouts per week.

❐ **Why It's Important:** Aerobic exercise trains the heart, lungs, and cardiovascular system to process and deliver oxygen more quickly and efficiently to every part of the body. As the heart muscle becomes stronger and more efficient, a larger amount of blood can be pumped with each stroke. Fewer strokes are then required to rapidly transport oxygen to all parts of the body.

STRENGTH TRAINING

❒ **What It Is:** Any activity that improves the condition of your muscles by making repeated movements against a force. Examples include lifting large or small weights, sit-ups, stair-stepping, and isometrics.

❒ **Why It's Important:** Strength training makes it easier to move heavy loads, whether they require carrying, pushing, pulling or lifting, as well as to participate in sports that require strength. The exercises are of various kinds. Some require changing the length of the muscle while maintaining the level of tension, others involve using special equipment to vary the tension in the muscles, and some entail contracting a muscle while maintaining its length.

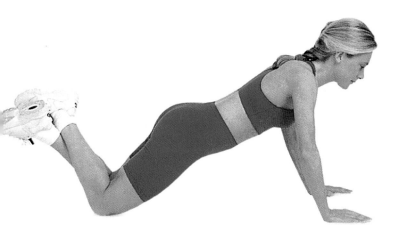

EATING SMART

A balanced diet is the foundation of good health. For proof, just read the numerous medical studies that link healthful eating with disease prevention and disease reversal. These same studies connect high fat intake, high sodium consumption, and diets with too much protein to numerous illnesses, including cancer, cardiovascular diseases, diverticular diseases, hypertension, and heart disease. But what exactly is a balanced diet? Generally speaking, it is a diet comprised of carbohydrates, dietary fiber, fat, protein, water, 13 vitamins, and 20 minerals. More specifically, it is a diet built around a wide variety of fruits, legumes, whole grains, and vegetables. Alcohol, animal protein, high-fat foods, high-sodium foods, highly-sugared foods, sodas, and processed foods are consumed sparingly, if at all.

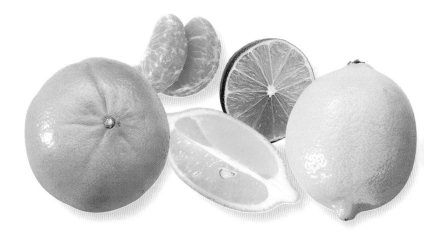

OMNIVOROUS

❏ **On the Menu:** Plant-based foods, dairy products, eggs, fish, seafood, red meats, organ meats, poultry.

❏ **Foods That Are Avoided:** None. Everything is fair game.

❏ **How Healthy Is It?** It depends. Someone who eats eggs, poultry or meat every day, chooses refined snacks over whole foods, and gets only one or two daily servings of fruits and vegetables will not be as healthy as a person who limits meat (the general dietary term for any "flesh foods," including poultry and fish) to two or three times a week, chooses water over soft drinks, and gets the recommended five or more daily servings of fruits and vegetables. Complaints about traditional omnivorous diets revolve around the diet's high level of cholesterol and saturated fat (found in animal-based foods), which increases one's risk of cancer, diabetes, heart disease, and obesity. However, an omnivorous diet can be a healthful one, provided thoughtful choices are made. To keep cholesterol and saturated fat to a minimum and nutrients to a maximum, eat five or more daily servings of fruits and vegetables, choose whole grains over refined grains, enjoy daily legume or soyfood protein sources, and limit the use of animal foods.

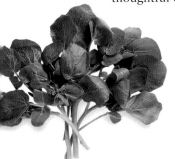

EATING SMART

MACROBIOTIC

❏ **On the Menu:** Plant-based foods, fish, very limited amounts of salt.

❏ **Foods That Are Avoided:** Dairy products, eggs, foods with artificial ingredients, hot spices, mass-produced foods, organ meats, peppers, potatoes, poultry, red meats, shellfish, warm drinks, refined foods.

❏ **How Healthy Is It?** Macrobiotics is based on a system created inn the early 1900s by Japanese philosopher George Ohsawa. The diet consists of 50 percent whole grains, 20 to 30 percent vegetables, and 5 to 10 percent beans, sea vegetables, and soy foods. The remainder of the diet is composed of white-meat fish, fruits, and nuts. The diet's low amounts of saturated fat, absence of processed foods, and emphasis on high-fiber foods, such as whole grains and vegetables, may promote cardiovascular health. Because soy and sea vegetables contain cancer-fighting compounds, macrobiotics is often recommended to help treat cancer. However, critics worry that the diet's limited variety of food can leave followers lacking in certain vitamins and important cancer-fighting phytonutrients.

PISCATORIAL

❏ **On the Menu:** Plant-based foods, dairy products, eggs, fish, seafood.

❏ **Foods That Are Avoided:** Red meats, organ meats, poultry.

❏ **How Healthy Is It?** Like an omnivorous diet, a piscatorial diet is as healthy as a person makes it. Individuals who eat high-fat and highly processed foods, fail to get the recommended daily number of vegetables and fruits, and eschew whole grains for processed grains will not enjoy optimum health. That said, individuals who are conscientious about eating a balanced, varied diet, and who limit fish and seafood intake to two or three times per week, can expect a lower risk of heart disease. Since many oily fish contain omega-3 fatty acids, eating oily fish in moderation has been found to help lower blood cholesterol. Be aware, however, that oily saltwater fish, such as shark, swordfish and tuna, have been found to carry mercury in their tissues; many health authorities recommend eating these varieties no more than once or twice a week. Also, due to overfishing, many fish species are now threatened, including bluefin tuna, Pacific perch, Chilean sea bass, Chinook salmon, and swordfish. For additional information on endangered fish, visit the University of Michigan's Endangered Species Update at www.umich.edu/~esuupdate, or the Fish and Wildlife Information Exchange at http://fwie.fe.vt.edu.

EATING SMART

VEGAN

❐ **On the Menu:** Plant-based foods.

❐ **Foods That Are Avoided:** Dairy, eggs, fish, seafood, red meats, organ meats, poultry. Also avoided are foods made by animals or processed with animal parts, such as gelatin, honey, marshmallows made with animal gelatin, white sugar processed with bone char.

❐ **How Healthy Is It?** A vegan (pronounced VEE-gun) diet can be extremely healthy. Like the vegetarian diet, a vegan diet has been shown by numerous studies to lower blood pressure and prevent heart disease. In addition, the high fiber intake cuts one's risk of diverticular disease and colon cancer. Yet because vegans do not eat dairy products or eggs, they must be more conscientious than vegetarians about either eating plant foods with vitamin B_{12} and vitamin D, or taking supplements of these nutrients.

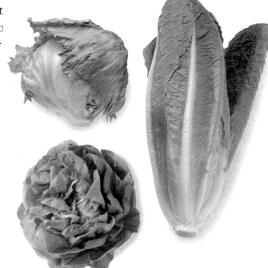

VEGETARIAN

❒ **On the Menu:** Plant-based foods, dairy, eggs.

❒ **Foods That Are Avoided:** Fish, gelatin, seafood, red meats, organ meats, poultry.

❒ **How Healthy Is It?** A vegetarian diet can be very healthy when done right. Fortunately, this isn't hard. Dietary science has debunked theories of "protein combining" popular in the 1960s and 1970s, leaving today's vegetarians to worry only about eating a wide variety of whole foods, including beans, fruits, grains, low-fat dairy products, nuts, soy foods, and vegetables. A varied daily diet insures enough protein, calcium, and other nutrients for vegetarians of all ages, including children, pregnant individuals, and the elderly. A well-chosen vegetarian eating plan has been shown by numerous studies to lower blood pressure, decrease one's risk of breast cancer, and prevent heart disease. In addition, the diet's high fiber levels cut the risk of diverticular disease and colon cancer.

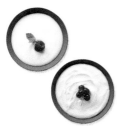

NUTRIENT KNOW-HOW

Vitamins and minerals are known collectively as nutrients. Name a body function, whether carbohydrate metabolism, nerve cell replication, or wound healing, and you'll find one or more of these nutrients at work. The best place to look for vitamins and minerals? In the food you eat every day. Indeed, if you eat a well-balanced diet there's a good chance you'll get all the nutrients your body needs. But if you are ill, pregnant, eat an inadequate diet, drink more than two alcoholic or caffeinated drinks per day,

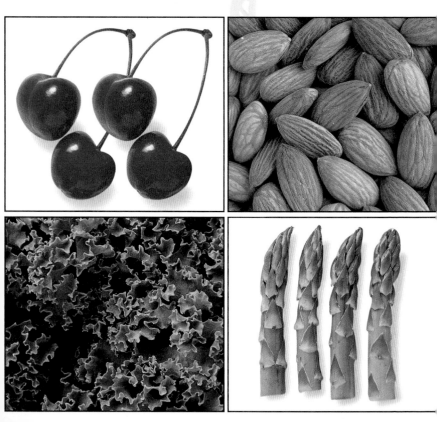

are under stress, are taking certain medications, or have difficulty absorbing certain nutrients, you may need to supplement your diet with one or more vitamins or minerals. Supplements generally come in tablet and capsule form, although some health food stores also carry liquid supplements. Whichever form you choose, doses are measured by weight in milligrams (mg); in micrograms (mcg); or in the universal standard known as international units (IU).

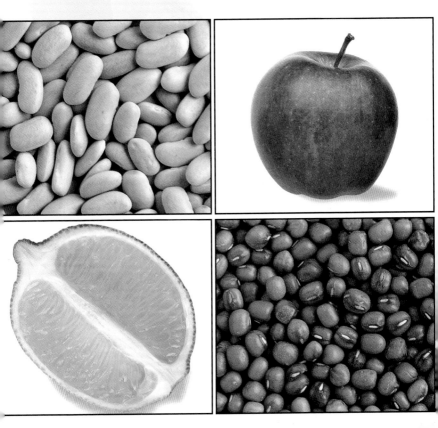

VITAMIN A

(beta carotene, retinol)

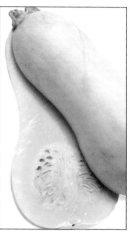

What It Does: Vitamin A is found in two forms: performed vitamin A, known as retinol, and provitamin A, called beta carotene. Retinol is found only in foods of animal origin. Beta carotene, a carotenoid, is a pigment found in plants. Beta carotene has a slight nutritional edge, boasting antioxidant properties and the ability to help lower harmful cholesterol levels. Regardless of the form, vitamin A is essential for good vision; promotes healthy skin, hair, and mucous membranes; stimulates wound healing; and is necessary for proper development of bones and teeth.

Recommended Daily Allowance: Men, 5,000 IU (or 3 mg beta carotene); women, 4,000 IU (or 2.4 mg beta carotene).

Food Sources: Orange and yellow fruits and vegetables, dark green leafy vegetables, whole milk, cream, butter, organ meats.

Toxic Dosage: When taken in excess of 10,000 IU daily, prolonged use of vitamin A supplements can cause abdominal pain, amenorrhea, dry skin, enlarged liver or spleen, hair loss, headaches, itching, joint pain, nausea, vision problems, vomiting.

Enemies: Antibiotics, cholesterol-lowering drugs, heavy laxative use.

Deficiency Symptoms: Because vitamin A is fat-soluble, it is stored in the body's fat for a long time, making deficiency uncommon. However, deficiency symptoms include dryness of the conjunctiva and cornea, frequent colds, insomnia, night blindness, reproductive difficulties, respiratory infections.

VITAMIN B_1

(thiamine)

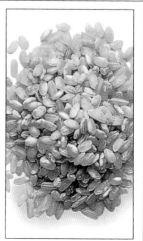

What It Does: Maintains normal nervous system functioning, helps metabolize carbohydrates, proteins, and fats; assists in blood formation and circulation; optimizes cognitive activity and brain function; regulates the body's appetite; protects the body from the degenerative effects of alcohol consumption, environmental pollution, and smoking.

Minimum Recommended Daily Allowance: Men, 1.5 mg; women, 1.1 mg.

Food Sources: Brewer's yeast, broccoli, brown rice, egg yolks, fish, legumes, peanuts, peas, pork, prunes, oatmeal, raisins, rice bran, soybeans, wheat germ, whole grains.

Toxic Dosage: There is no know toxicity level for vitamin B_1.

Enemies: Antibiotics, a diet high in simple carbohydrates, heavy physical exertion, oral contraceptives, sulfa drugs.

Deficiency Symptoms: Appetite loss, confusion, fatigue, heart arrhythmia, nausea, mood swings. Severe deficiency can lead to beriberi, a crippling disease characterized by convulsions, diarrhea, edema, gastrointestinal problems, heart failure, mental confusion, nerve damage, paralysis, severe weight loss.

VITAMIN B₂

(riboflavin, vitamin G)
What It Does: Helps metabolize carbohydrates, fats, and proteins; allows skin, nail, and hair tissues to utilize oxygen; aids in red blood cell formation and antibody production; promotes cell respiration; maintains proper nerve function, eyes, and adrenal glands.
Minimum Recommended Daily Allowance: Men, 1.7 mg; women, 1.3 mg; pregnant women, 1.6 mg.
Food Sources: Cheese, egg yolks, fish, legumes, milk, poultry, spinach, whole grains, yogurt.
Toxic Dosage: There is no known toxicity level for this vitamin, although nervousness and rapid heartbeat have been reported with daily dosages of 10 mg.
Enemies: Alcohol, oral contraceptives, strenuous exercise.
Deficiency Symptoms: Cracks at the corners of the mouth, dermatitis, dizziness, hair loss, insomnia, itchy or burning eyes, light sensitivity, mouth sores, impaired thinking, inflammation of the tongue, rashes.

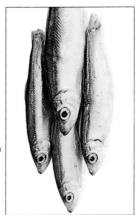

VITAMIN B₅

(pantothenic acid)
What It Does: Helps produce adrenal hormones, antibodies, and various neurotransmitters; reduces skin inflammation; speeds healing of wounds; helps convert food to energy.
Minimum Recommended Daily Allowance: 4 mg.
Food Sources: Beef, eggs, beans, brown rice, corn, lentils, mushrooms, nuts, peas, pork, saltwater fish, sweet potatoes.
Toxic Dosages: There is no known toxicity level for this vitamin; however, doses above 10 mg can cause diarrhea in some individuals.
Deficiency Symptoms: Vitamin B₅ deficiency is extremely rare and is likely to occur only with starvation.

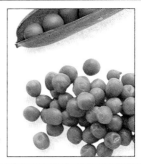

VITAMIN B₆

(pyridoxine)
What It Does: Involved in more bodily functions than nearly any other nutrient. It helps the body metabolize carbohydrates, fats and proteins; supports immune function; helps build red blood cells; assists in transmission of nerve impulses; maintains the body's sodium and potassium balance; helps synthesize RNA and DNA.
Minimum Recommended Daily Allowance: Men, 2 mg; women, 1.6 mg; pregnant women, 2.2 mg.
Food Sources: Avocados, bananas, beans, blackstrap molasses, brown rice, carrots, corn, fish, nuts, sunflower seeds.
Toxic Dosage: Levels of 2,000 to 5,000 mg can cause numbness in the hands and feet, and insomnia.
Deficiency Symptoms: Vitamin B₆ deficiency is rare. Symptoms include depression, fatigue, flaky skin, headaches, insomnia, irritability, muscle weakness, nausea.

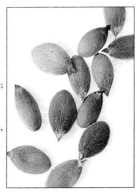

VITAMIN B$_{12}$

(cobalamin)

What It Does: Regulates formation of red blood cells, helps the body utilize iron; converts carbohydrates, fats, and proteins into energy; aids in cellular formation and cellular longevity; prevents nerve damage; maintains fertility; promotes normal growth.

Minimum Recommended Daily Allowance: Adults, 2 mg; pregnant women, 2.2 mg.

Food Sources: Brewer's yeast, dairy products, eggs, organ meats, seafood, sea vegetables, tempeh.

Toxic Dosage: There is no known toxicity level for vitamin B$_{12}$.

Enemies: Anticoagulant drugs, anti gout medication, potassium supplements.

Deficiency Symptoms: While deficiency is rare, individuals who do not eat animal products are at risk unless they fortify their diets with plant-sources such as brewer's yeast and sea vegetables. Symptoms include back pain, body odor, constipation, dizziness, fatigue, moodiness, numbness and tingling in the arms and legs, ringing in the ears, muscle weakness, tongue inflammation, weight loss. Severe deficiency can lead to pernicious anemia, characterized by abdominal pain, stiffness in the arms and legs, a tendency to bleed, yellowish cast to the skin, permanent nerve damage, death.

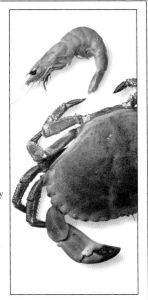

VITAMIN C

(ascorbic acid)

What It Does: Protects against pollution and infection, enhances immunity; aids in growth and repair of both bone and tissue by helping the body produce collagen; maintains adrenal gland function; helps the body absorb iron; aids in production of antistress hormones; reduces cholesterol levels; lowers high blood pressure; prevents artherosclerosis.

Minimum Recommended Daily Allowance: Adults, 60 mg; pregnant women, 70 mg.

Food Sources: Berries, cantaloupe, citrus fruits, broccoli, leafy greens, mangoes, papayas, peppers, persimmons, pineapple, tomatoes.

Toxic Dosage: Doses larger than 10,000 mg can cause diarrhea, stomach irritation, or increased kidney stone formation. **Enemies:** Alcohol, analgesics, antidepressants, anticoagulants, oral contraceptives, smoking, steroids.

Deficiency Symptoms: Bleeding gums, easy bruising, fatigue, reduced resistance to colds and other infections, slow healing of wounds, weight loss. Severe deficiency can lead to scurvy, a sometimes-fatal disease characterized by aching bones, muscle weakness, and swollen and bleeding gums.

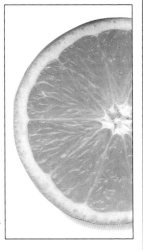

VITAMIN D

(calciferol, ergosterol)

What It Does: Helps the body utilize calcium and phosphorus; promotes normal development of bones and teeth; assists in thyroid function; maintains normal blood clotting; helps regulate heartbeat, nerve function, and muscle contraction.

Minimum Recommended Daily Allowance: Adults, 200 IU (5 mcg); pregnant women, 400 IU (10 mcg).

Food Sources: Dandelion greens, dairy products, eggs, fatty saltwater fish, parsley, sweet potatoes, vegetable oils.

Toxic Dosage: Daily doses higher than 400 IU can lead to raised blood calcium levels and calcium deposits of the heart, liver, and kidney.

Enemies: Antacids, cholesterol-lowering drugs, cortisone drugs.

Deficiency Symptoms: The body naturally manufactures about 200 IU of vitamin D when exposed to ten minutes of ultraviolet light, making deficiency rare. Symptoms include bone weakening, diarrhea, insomnia, muscle twitches, vision disturbances. Severe deficiency can lead to rickets, a disease that results in bone defects such as bowlegs and knock-knees.

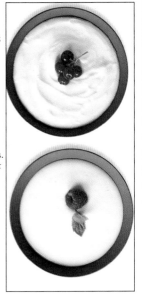

VITAMIN E

(tocopherol)

What It Does: Prevents unstable molecules known as free radicals from damaging cells and tissue; accelerates wound healing; protects lung tissue from inhaled pollutants; aids in functioning of the immune system; endocrine system, and sex glands; improves circulation; promotes normal blood clotting.

Minimum Recommended Daily Allowance: Men, 15 IU (10 mg); women, 12 IU (8 mg); pregnant women, 15 IU (10 mg).

Food Sources: Avocados, dark green leafy vegetables, eggs, legumes, nuts, organ meats, seafood, seeds, soybeans.

Toxic Dosage: Although there is no established toxicity level of vitamin E, the vitamin has blood-thinning properties; individuals who are taking anticoagulant medications or have clotting deficiencies should avoid vitamin E.

Enemies: High temperatures and overcooking reduce vitamin E levels in food.

Deficiency Symptoms: Vitamin E deficiency is rare. Deficiency symptoms include fluid retention, infertility, miscarriage, muscle degeneration.

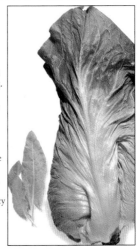

CALCIUM

What It Does: Necessary for the growth and maintenance of bones, teeth, and healthy gums; maintains normal blood pressure normal; may reduce risk of heart disease; enables muscles, including the heart, to contract; is essential for normal blood clotting; needed for proper nerve impulse transmission; maintains connective tissue; helps prevent rickets and osteoporosis.

Minimum Recommended Daily Allowance: Adults, 800 mg; pregnant women, 1,200 mg.

Food Sources: Asparagus, cruciferous vegetables, dairy products, dark leafy vegetables, figs, legumes, nuts, oats, prunes, salmon with bones, sardines with bones, seeds, soybeans, tempeh, tofu.

Toxic Dosage: Daily intake of 2,000 mg or more can lead to constipation, calcium deposits in the soft tissue, urinary tract infections, and possible interference with the body's absorption of zinc.

Enemies: Alcohol, caffeine, excessive sugar intake, high-protein diet, high sodium intake, inadequate levels of vitamin D, soft drinks containing phosphorous.

Deficiency Symptoms: Aching joints, brittle nails, eczema, elevated blood cholesterol, heart palpitations, hypertension, insomnia, muscle cramps, nervousness, pallor, tooth decay.

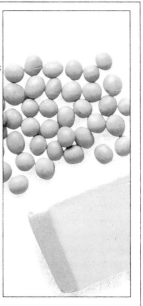

IRON

What It Does: Aids in the production of hemoglobin (the protein in red blood cells that transports oxygen from the lungs to the body's tissue) and myoglobin (a protein that provides extra fuel to muscles during exertion); helps maintain healthy immune system; is important for growth.

Minimum Recommended Daily Allowance: Men, 10 mg; women, 15 mg; pregnant women, 30 mg.

Food Sources: Beef, blackstrap molasses, brewer's yeast, dark green vegetables, dried fruit, legumes, nuts, organ meats, sea vegetables, seeds, soybeans, tempeh, whole grains.

Toxic Dosage: Iron should not be taken in excess of 35 mg daily without a doctor's recommendation. In high doses, iron cam cause diarrhea, dizziness, fatigue, headaches, stomach-aches, weakened pulse. Excess iron inhibits the absorption of phosphorus and vitamin E, interferes with immune function, and has been associated with cancer, cirrhosis, heart disease.

Enemies: Antacids, caffeine, tetracycline, iron absorption, excessive menstrual bleeding, long-term illness, an ulcer.

Deficiency Symptoms: Anemia, brittle hair, difficulty swallowing, dizziness, fatigue, hair loss, irritability, nervousness, pallor, ridges on the nails, sensitivity to cold, slowed mental reactions.

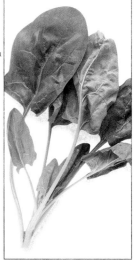

MAGNESIUM

What It Does: Plays a role in formation of bone; protects arterial linings from stress caused by sudden blood pressure; helps body metabolize carbohydrates and minerals; assists in building proteins; helps maintain healthy bones and teeth; reduces one's risk of developing osteoporosis.
Minimum Recommended Daily Allowance: Men, 350 mg; women, 280 mg; pregnant women, 320 mg.
Food Sources: Apples, apricots, avocados, bananas, blackstrap molasses, brewer's yeast. brown rice, cantaloupe, dairy products, figs, garlic, green leafy vegetables, legumes, nuts.
Toxic Dosage: Daily doses over 3,000 mg can lead to diarrhea, fatigue, muscle weakness, and in extreme cases, severely depressed heart rate and blood pressure, shallow breathing, loss of reflexes and coma.
Enemies: Alcohol, diuretics, high-fat intake, high-protein diet.
Deficiency Symptoms: Though deficiency is rare, symptoms include disorientation, heart palpitations, listlessness, muscle weakness.

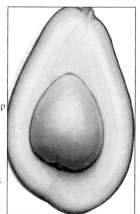

POTASSIUM

What It Does: Maintains a healthy nervous system and regular heart rhythm; helps prevent stroke; aids in proper muscle contractions; controls the body's water balance; assists chemical reactions within cells; aids in the transmission of electrochemical impulses; maintains stable blood pressure; required for protein synthesis, carbohydrate metabolism, and insulin secretion by the pancreas.
Minimum Recommended Daily Allowance: Adults, 2,000 mg.
Food Sources: Apricots, avocados, bananas, blackstrap molasses, brewer's yeast, brown rice, citrus fruits, dairy.
Toxic Dosage: Should not be taken in excess of 18 grams.

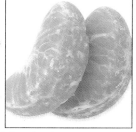

Enemies: Diarrhea, diuretics, caffeine use, heavy perspiration, kidney disorders, tobacco use.
Deficiency Symptoms: Chills, dry skin, constipation, depression, diminished reflexes, edema, headaches, insatiable thirst, fluctuations in heartbeat, nervousness, respiratory distress.

ZINC

What It Does: Contributes to a wide range of bodily processes. Aids in cell respiration; assists in bone development; helps energy metabolism, promotes wound healing; regulates heart rate and blood pressure; helps liver remove toxic substances, such as alcohol, from the body.
Minimum Recommended Daily Allowance: Adults, 15 mg; pregnant women, 30 mg.
Food Sources: Brewer's yeast, cheese, egg yolks, lamb, legumes, mushrooms, nuts, organ meats, sea food, sea vegetables, seeds.
Toxic Dosage: Do not take more than 100 mg of zinc daily. In doses this high, zinc can depress the immune system.
Deficiency Symptoms: Appetite loss, dermatitis, fatigue, impaired wound healing, loss of taste, white streaks on the nails.

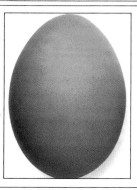

INDEX

ABOUT THE AUTHOR

Stephanie Pedersen is a writer and editor who specializes in the area of health. Her articles have appeared in numerous publications, including *American Woman, Sassy, Teen, Weight Watchers* and *Woman's World*. She has also co-written *What Your Cat is Trying to Tell You: A Head-to-Tail Guide to Your Cat's Symptoms and Their Solutions* and *What Your Dog is Trying to Tell You: A Head-to-Tail Guide to Your Dog's Symptoms and Their Solutions*, both published by St. Martin's Press. She currently resides in New York City.

Picture Credits: Steve Gorton, David Murray, Dave King, Martin Norris, Philip Gatward, Andy Crawford, Philip Dowell, Clive Streeter, Peter Chadwick, Tim Ridley, Andrew Whittack, Martin Cameron

DORLING KINDERSLEY PUBLISHING, INC.
www.dk.com

Published in the United States by
Dorling Kindersley Publishing, Inc.
95 Madison Avenue • New York, New York 10016

Copyright © 2000 by Dorling Kindersley Publishing, Inc.

Editorial Director: LaVonne Carlson
Editors: Nancy Burke, Barbara Minton, Connie Robinson
Designer: Carol Wells
Cover Designer: Gus Yoo

Library of Congress Cataloging-in-Publication Data is available upon request.
ISBN: 0-7894-5198-0